AWAKENING TO HEALTH

...DISCOVERING THE TRUTH

Ron Garner

Foreword by
Dr. Robert Rowe, DC

Library and Archives Canada Publication Data

Garner, Ron 1938 –

AWAKENING TO HEALTH

Subtitle: Discovering the TRUTH

Book ISBN: 978-0-9688362-8-6

eBook ISBN: 978-0-9688362-9-3

1. Health 2. Disease 3. Garner, Ron. Title

Publisher: Independent

Cover Design: Ron Garner

Cover Model: Amanda Beal

Cover Photo: Blaise Enright

Website: http://www.awakeningtohealth.ca

DISCLAIMER

The author, Ron Garner, is not a doctor or healthcare practitioner. He does not have clients, and is not available to advise people about their specific health problems.

The information presented here is the result of his research and efforts to correct his own health challenges that plagued him since he was a child, and to understand the truth about how the human body is designed to function in health.

This material is presented as information only. What you do with it is your decision and responsibility.

Neither the author nor publisher shall be liable or responsible for any loss or damage allegedly arising from any information or suggestion in this book/course.

TABLE OF CONTENTS

ABOUT THE AUTHOR and this information

Ron Garner, BEd, MSc, is the award-winning author of *Conscious Health* and lives in British Columbia Canada. Since his retirement from the educational field in 1996 he has devoted his time to discovering how we can live free of disease. He is a passionate seeker of the truth in all matters affecting our society and environments.

Since he was a very young child Ron suffered from health problems – eczema, allergies, asthma, digestive complaints and bowel issues. In his fifties he realized that pharmaceutical medications were not bringing back the health he saw in others. He began to search for answers in the natural health field. Ron discovered that there is no quick fix – learning and renewal of health takes time and perseverance. Over the past thirty years he has been able to sort through the confusion and discover teachings of the most brilliant minds regarding how our bodies are designed to operate and what they require to function efficiently.

This book/course, *Awakening to Health*, is the distillation of the best and most effective natural health teachings he has discovered. It contains the shortest but clear explanation regarding why we get sick and how we can be well. While he has made personal health gains over the years, the most impressive were made during this last year after he fully embraced Dr. Robert O Young's discovery regarding the new biology of digestion. At 86 years now, he is delighted to enjoy increased energy, a renewed sense of well-being and a strong immune system with all its benefits. His friends are surprised at his level of energy and health for his age.

Ron shares this knowledge with others to help as many as possible break free of the conditioning of helplessness and dependence that pervades our world societies regarding sickness and disease. Knowledge is power when it is applied.

Our world has become scary and, in many ways, dangerous. The air, water, food, and medicines have been laced with ingredients harmful to all life. To survive, we need to be knowledgeable independent thinkers who ask questions and learn to take care of ourselves. We must accept personal responsibility for our own well-being.

The purpose of this material is to unveil the truth about how the human body operates and open the door of health freedom for everyone. All the reader needs are the desire to learn and the will to apply it to their own life.

When you have completed this book/course, you will realize that health is a choice…but so is disease. They both depend on your decision to either work with or against your body's innate wisdom to produce health.

First, we must gain knowledge, so let's proceed.

FOREWORD

In 1975 I graduated from the Canadian Memorial Chiropractic College and was ready to relieve the unnecessary pain and suffering of the world…only to find that there was much more to learn.

We were given many hours of biochemistry and nutrition instruction to understand the digestive processes and need for different food components, as well as the role of vitamins and minerals. However, I soon realized that putting this information into use for patients with complicated problems needed a lot more study.

I spent many years following health gurus regarding what we should eat. Each one had their own opinion. I eventually realized that every person, and patient, is different.

The world is focused on treating disease and except for exercise, most people are just chasing disease symptoms, not correcting the root cause.

I spent a lot of time studying naturopathic medicine in the early 1980's and noticed each instructor had a favorite way of diagnosing and treating patients. Sorting it all out was a challenge. In the mid 1980's I studied with Dr. George Goodheart and his approach using muscle testing to discover deficiencies in the body.

I also spent a lot of time studying and using functional medicine, with good results. However, it was again focused on evaluating the disease condition of the body and using natural approaches to help the body.

I met Ron Garner around 2006 and read his book *Conscious Health*, an award-winning book, on understanding what health is and what contributes to and what destroys it. This was the information I had been searching for, for many years because it focused on health not disease. This book should have been required reading in all the alternative health school programs. I was now on a better path to understanding that building a healthy body was not only possible but within reach of everyone. As a matter of fact, it was the only way to true health.

Ron's book didn't include western medicine because their focus is on disease treatment. Sometimes treatment is necessary to save lives, but after the life is saved the journey to optimal natural health should start.

Ron has recovered his own health after serious health challenges early in his life and has spent years studying the greats in the natural health field. He has been relentless in putting everything to the test and never giving up. As a result, he has refined it all to a simple approach based on optimal body chemistry and how to attain it.

The body has all it needs to be healthy if it is allowed to do its job with balanced body chemistry.

His new book *Awakening to Health* puts it in simple terms on how to measure the state of one's body chemistry and how to use simple steps to optimize it.

Just following this simple process over time, you can rise to a higher state of health and have a better life.

The first step in an exercise program is getting up and just starting. The first step toward improved health is just starting to change what you put in your mouth.

Have a great journey in optimizing your body chemistry and having a better life.

Dr. Robert Rowe, DC

INTRODUCTION

Nothing in life is to be feared; it is only to be
understood. Now is the time to understand
more so that we may fear less.
...Marie Curie

Why I Wrote This Book

Simply stated... to help people understand how to live free of disease. It is written to be a straight-to-the-point, easy-to-read, and understandable reference for gaining full knowledge to enable you to take control of your health.

Awakening

Awakening is defined as the act of waking up, or no longer sleeping. It is becoming aware of what is happening around and to us. It is not simply accepting what some person or authority tells us is truth; it is observing, learning and thinking to determine our own perception of the actual reality of things so we can make decisions in our own best interests.

Awakening to health means developing awareness of the illusion created for us that health is so difficult to understand we need some medical authority to keep us healthy. But, much of what we have been conditioned to believe is not true. The purpose of this book, actually a short learning course, is to give you knowledge about how your body operates so you can help it create the vibrant health it was designed to do.

What Doctors Don't Know

As the author, I have no desire or intention to denigrate doctors because I am sure most of them are well-meaning and sincere in their desire to help people. Allopathic trauma care is excellent, but true health care for illness and disease conditions is another matter.

On their way to being licensed to practice medicine, all doctors spend years studying and learning a great amount of information. However, they are not free to pursue subjects outside the boundaries of what is prescribed by their schools nor, after they graduate, are they free to use treatment modalities not sanctioned by their medical associations. They are trained to follow rules, but not necessarily educated about how to help the human body heal itself naturally.

The training of doctors in medical schools is designed to support an industry that makes large sums of money. Doctors work in a for-profit system. Temporary relief of illness symptoms using pharmaceutical drugs and scheduling repeat visits to doctors and specialists are the goals, not permanent natural healing of ailments based on correcting the cause of health problems. They have had almost no education regarding nutrition or detoxification.

There are two main components critical to good health most doctors, both allopathic and naturopathic, do not understand or apply in their practices:

1. They do not know the basic cause of disease. When you read in a doctor's PDR (Physician's Desk Reference) about specific disease conditions, you will typically find the phrase: "cause unknown." If you don't know the cause of a problem, how can you fix it?

2. Doctors are not taught complete understanding of how the human body operates. Specifically, they have not learned how the body's cellular wastes are eliminated by its extensive lymphatic sewer system.

An Analogy

Doctors are trained to concentrate on blood analysis but totally ignore the lymphatic system. This is equivalent to a person caring for their car by always keeping it washed and the gas tank full but never changing the oil or filters. Waste products from fuel combustion eventually build up to cause problems with the car's engine. Sludge takes its inevitable toll. The same thing happens in the human body.

Why Doctors Don't Know

The reason doctors don't know the basic cause of why the human body develops disease, and how it works naturally to keep itself healthy, stems from the Flexner Report on Medical Education in the United States and Canada, published in 1910. This large study report was written by Abraham Flexner, who was sponsored and financed by the Carnegie Foundation and John D. Rockefeller, after visiting and interviewing the staff of 155 medical schools in the US and Canada. "It elevated the importance of German educational methods in the teaching of medicine."[1]

In her article, *The Flexner Report: How John D. Rockefeller Used the AMA to Take Over Western Medicine*[2], Makia Freeman outlines the main considerations and outcomes regarding this report:

- Rockefeller had made a massive fortune with Standard Oil and was setting his sights on gaining a monopoly in the drug and pharmaceutical industry. However, he had to get rid of the competition, which consisted of natural non-allopathic healing modalities – naturopathy, homeopathy, eclectic medicine (botanical and herbal medicine), holistic medicine etc.

- Its main objective was the standardization of medical education by concluding that there were too many doctors and medical schools in America.

- Rockefeller used his control of the media to generate public outcry at the findings of the report...which ultimately led Congress to declare the AMA (American Medical Association) the only body with the right to grant medical school licenses in the United States.

- After the Flexner Report, the AMA only endorsed schools with a drug-based curriculum. It didn't take long before non-allopathic schools fell by the wayside due to lack of funding.

Impact on Alternative Medicine

"Flexner clearly doubted the scientific validity of all forms of medicine other than that based on scientific research, deeming any approach to medicine that did not advocate the use of treatments such as vaccines to prevent and cure illness as tantamount to quackery and charlatanism. Medical schools that offered training in various disciplines including electromagnetic field therapy, phototherapy, eclectic medicine, physiomedicalism, naturopathy, and homeopathy, were told either to drop these courses from their curriculum or lose their

---

[1] www.cancertutor.com, January 9, 2019

[2] Freeman, Makia, The Flexner Report: How John D. Rockefeller Used the AMA to Take Over Western Medicine,https://thefreedomarticles.com/flexner-report-rockefeller-ama-takeover/, 2012 and 2015

accreditation and underwriting support. A few schools resisted for a time, but eventually most complied with the Report or shut their doors."[3]

What the Flexner Report effectively did was to "create a culture that enabled the monetization of medicine" and "paved the way for (the) overthrow of whole-body health by making scientific research and training alone the only desirable and credible approach to human wellness."[4]

The plan to take over western medicine and shape beliefs about health was masterfully conceived and implemented. The result has been almost total mind-control and market-harvesting of an unsuspecting and uneducated public regarding the truths about health and disease.

---

3 www.en.wikipedia.org/wiki/Flexner_Report
4 www.principia-scientific.org/how-the-flexner-report-hijacked-natural-medicine/,cancertutor.com, January 9, 2019.
202

SECTION 1: What is Disease?

We have been taught to believe disease is caused by a germ, bacteria, or virus that attacks our body from the outside, but this is not true. In fact, almost all so-called diseases develop due to toxic pollution of our internal fluids. This causes an alteration of the body's natural chemical and electrical balances, both of which are closely related. In this book/course you will learn what these causes are and how to help your body return to its natural balance, or homeostasis.

More specifically stated, disease symptoms are the manifestation of a state of dis-ease, dis-comfort, or inefficient operation of one or more internal organs and glands. They are caused by retained pollutants - wastes, that in most cases we can help the body eliminate by simple changes in our lifestyle.

Disease begins when any cell
loses its ability to function efficiency.

Aren't there many diseases?

Actually NO! There are many *symptoms* of dis-ease the body presents, depending on the organ, gland, or system that is out of nutritional or chemical balance. The allopathic and pharmaceutically-based medical system would have us believe there are hundreds of diseases. Disease is made to seem so complex, scary, and beyond our ability to understand that we need doctors to help us back to health, often with the use of drug prescriptions. But this is not true and not always necessary because disease and health are simple to understand, as you will soon discover. You will learn to look at health from a natural point of view of what the human body requires in order to correct imbalances and return to normal functioning and vibrant health.

What is a doctor?

The original meaning of 'doctor' was 'teacher' – one who teaches others how to be healthy. Has this been your experience with doctors? In most cases probably not, because in their training doctors spend very few hours learning how nutrition affects health. They are trained under a pharmaceutically-based curriculum and are required to follow directives of their professional medical associations.

Are all drugs bad?

Absolutely not! In times of crisis some drugs can save lives. This author's life was saved twice by antibiotics to overcome blood poisoning. However, drugs used must have a safety record and should only be used temporarily until the crisis is over.

Health-care or Disease-care?

The present medical system advertises under the name of *healthcare*, but people go to a doctor because they don't feel well – they have a symptom or feeling of illness, a dis-ease in their body. So, the medical system actually provides a *disease-care* service that treats symptoms but does not focus on causes to restore health. In most cases, drugs mask symptoms for temporary relief but do not contribute to making the body stronger. We have been misled to believe it is about health. True healthcare focuses on correcting deficiencies and imbalances so the body can heal itself.

Final thought

One does not need a degree to gain an understanding of how to be healthy. We just need to be willing to learn and apply it to our life. That's what this book/course is all about.

 Why Disease Happens

Disease happens when your body is not given the nutrition it needs to produce healthy cells and efficiently eliminate wastes. Healthy cells are chemically alkaline and electrically charged with voltage. When cells are alkaline, voltage is also strong.

The body is alkaline by design and acidic by function. Just as a car engine operates by burning fuel and producing waste as exhaust, your body operates in the same way. But if waste products are allowed to build up, malfunction or disease (dis-ease) begins to happen. Waste products are acidic. Acids are corrosive; they burn and damage tissues, weaken cellular function and lead to lower levels of oxygen, energy, and a weakened immune system.

The most critical areas that become congested by waste products are the colon and kidneys. As this happens, acids are retained, causing dis-ease or lack of function in various body areas. All disease symptoms are the result of acid build-up, called acidosis. As acidosis increases, oxygen and voltage in cells decrease.

- The cleaner your internal organs are, the more efficiently your body functions.
- The more consistently alkaline and electrically-alive your intake of food is, the healthier your cells will be.

The cause of all disease

As stated by Dr. Robert O Young, world-renowned microscopy expert and author of the excellent book *The pH Miracle*: *"The cause of all disease, except for having something injected by a needle, is acidosis."* Acids are produced within the body as waste from cellular metabolism
and digestive processing of foods and beverages. When these are excessive, eliminative organs – especially the colon and kidneys - become congested, causing wastes to be retained in inflamed body tissues. Inflammation is another word for acidosis. Damage to tissues and weakening of organ functions begin to happen.

What about parasites?

Parasites do not cause disease, but are a secondary problem. All parasites are scavengers – they are part of nature's clean-up crew to reduce waste buildup. If a body is internally clean and healthy, there is little waste - oxygen levels are high and there is no suitable environment to support parasites. You can take herbs to kill parasites, but if you do not also address your internal acidic waste problem, parasites will return.

What can you do to correct or avoid the development of disease?

Take responsibility for your own health! You are the change you need to see.

Understand This…

There is no drug, supplement, healer, modality, or technology that will permanently transform and heal you without you taking personal responsibility for correcting what allowed the health problem to be created in the first place. That requires you to change some lifestyle practices to return your body to its natural internal acid/alkaline balance.

 Health is Simple

The cause of disease is made to seem complex but it is not, because as Dr. Robert Morse explains in his book, *The Detox Miracle Sourcebook*…

*"There are only two sides to chemistry,
and there are only two major fluids in a cell."*

Only Two Sides to Chemistry – Acid and Alkaline

"Disease happens on the acid side of chemistry because acids are corrosive; they burn. Health is maintained on the alkaline side of chemistry because blood must be kept slightly alkaline with a pH as near as possible to 7.4. A prolonged acidic lifestyle moves the blood pH lower, forcing the body to withdraw alkaline minerals, mainly calcium, from its vessel walls and connective tissues to maintain a balanced and stable blood pH. This causes corrosion, weakening of connective tissues, and deterioration of arteries, veins, glands and organs."

Two Major Fluids in a Cell – Blood and Lymph

*"Every single part of the body is made up of
a bunch of cells and two fluids."*
- Dr. Robert Morse

Quoting from Dr. Morse, "We have approximately one hundred trillion cells in our body. Every cell must be nourished, and every cell must eliminate its metabolic wastes. Blood brings nourishment to the cells and lymph takes cellular wastes away. Approximately 25% of cellular fluid is slightly alkaline blood; the other 75% is mostly lymph that collects acidic wastes."

In other words, each cell has a kitchen system and a sewage system. If the sewer system, called the lymphatic system, is unable to eliminate wastes efficiently through the kidneys it begins to congest and constipate, causing acids to be retained and stored in the body. When this happens, the acid-laden lymph corrodes tissues and lowers oxygen levels in these areas, causing the form and function of cells to change. This is how disease conditions develop. That's all there is to it. It is not complicated.

The Keys to Health

Considering the simplicity of understanding acid/alkaline and blood/lymph, the solution to creating health and eliminating disease conditions in the body is to concentrate on detoxification and alkalization. This is always the remedy.

SECTION 4: How to Maximize Electrical Energy in Your Body

When we are healthy, we feel strong and full of energy. The human body was designed to generate and store energy (electrons) from:

1. Eating living food
2. Drinking structured alkaline water
3. Breathing clean air
4. Doing moderate exercise. Muscles are piezoelectric – they generate electrical energy through movement.
5. Making direct contact with the earth. The earth's Schumann Resonance vibrates at the frequency of 7.83 Hz. Scientific studies have shown that the human brain reaches its full potential for health and wellness when it vibrates with the same frequency as the earth. You can also buy an earthing sheet for your bed to enjoy contact with this earth energy as you sleep.
6. Sunshine
7. Getting 7 or 8 hours of deep, restful sleep each night.

Electron Donors and Stealers

Foods and beverages are either electron donors or electron stealers, according to their alkalinity or acidity. They either add to or subtract from, the body's electrical voltage. Raw foods are electron donors. Cooked and processed foods are electron stealers.

For further understanding of the electrical nature of the human body, check out the work of Dr. Jerry Tennant, author of the book *Healing is Voltage*.

Stimulating Foods Put Strain on the Adrenal Glands   It can be difficult to understand why foods that make us feel good, such as coffee, meat, and alcohol, are causing harm to the body. The reason is because the body sees them as harmful and wants to eliminate them quickly. To do this, it instructs the adrenal glands to secrete adrenaline to speed up metabolism. As this happens, we feel a burst of energy, but this comes at a cost; over time it is tiring. Consumption of stimulants lowers adrenal gland strength and body vitality. The primary cause of low energy is acid/alkaline imbalance, which leads to weakened adrenal glands.

When Over-Exercising can be Harmful

While muscle movement improves blood circulation and generates electrical energy, it also produces a waste product called lactic acid which must be cleared from the body. Lactic acid is approximately 4000 to 5000 times more acidic than water with a neutral pH of 7.0.

For someone whose body is acidic, high intensity exercise just adds to their problem because it produces more acid than their body is able to eliminate. As stated in Section 2, all disease symptoms are the result of acid build-up, called acidosis.

Therefore, one should stay with moderate exercise until they have returned their body to a healthy acid-alkaline balance.

SECTION 5: How to Reverse the Disease Process

Simply explained, this is done by giving your body what it needs to be internally clean and become alkaline.

Stop doing the wrong things, and start doing the right things.

1. Detoxify the main organs of elimination: colon, kidneys, skin.
2. Incorporate foods and supplements into your diet to alkalize your body and assist with detoxifying your organs and tissues.
3. Eliminate, or at least minimize, acid-producing foods and beverages.
4. Maximize living, electrically alive, alkaline fruits and vegetables in your diet.
5. Do moderate exercise such as walking, cycling, rebounding, for 20 to 30 minutes each day to increase blood circulation, move lymph, and generate electrical energy.
6. Incorporate intermittent fasting into your health practices.

In short, work to detoxify and bring acid/alkaline balance into the body. What follows will be increased oxygen, electro-magnetic energy, and feelings of well-being.

SECTION 6: Detoxification - How to Flush out Toxins Stored in the Body

Detoxification is the process of removing stored wastes and toxic acids. The body naturally and periodically detoxifies by bringing on colds and flues. But if toxic diet and lifestyle practices are not corrected, acids continue to accumulate in organs, glands, and tissues.

Wastes from cellular metabolism and digestion become distributed throughout the body. However, if we concentrate on helping the main organs of elimination do their job, health creation tends to take care of itself. The main organs of elimination to concentrate on are the colon, kidneys, and skin. As you progress further on this journey, liver cleanses can bring additional benefits.

Keys to Detoxification

1. Introduce more, preferably organic, raw fruits and vegetables into the diet
2. Cleanse the colon. This can be assisted by using enemas, colonic irrigations, and herbal cleansers such as *Herb Cocktail* from avenaoriginals.com. "OxyPowder" is another great product.
3. Make sure the kidneys are filtering. Pee in a jar to see if there is fine sediment, which is cellular waste. If not, the kidneys may be congested. Then, one may help them to filter by using:
   - Kidney and adrenal herbs
   - Fasting. Most effective is dry fasting. (One day of dry fasting is equivalent to three days of water fasting. Check out the work of Russian Dr. Sergei Filonov.
4. Skin health. Skin problems are a clear sign the body requires detoxification. When the kidneys become congested, the body resorts to moving wastes through the skin. (The skin is also referred to as the third kidney.) To help the skin more effectively remove wastes you can:
   - Move to a more raw, alkaline diet

- Minimize the use of lotions that clog pores
- Do dry skin brushing
- Do mild to moderate exercise to promote sweating
- Have hot and cold alternating showers
- Take 30-minute bath soaks in very warm water with one or a combination of sea salt, Epsom salts, and aluminum-free baking soda
- Take regular saunas

 Understanding pH

The pH (hydrogen ion concentration) scale, used to measure acid and alkaline strength, ranges from 0 to 14. Zero is most acidic and 14 most alkaline; 7 is neutral. Balanced liquids have a pH of 7. The body *must* maintain a blood pH as close as possible to an alkaline level of 7.365. It does whatever is necessary to keep blood pH constant. If blood pH falls to 7.1 the body goes into a coma, and at pH 6.9 the body dies.

The pH scale for acid-alkaline is similar to the Richter scale for measuring the intensity of earthquakes; they are both measures of exponential change. Each one-point change in the scale results in a tenfold change in strength. For example, a reading of pH 6.0 indicates an effective acid strength of ten (10), while an acid at pH 5.0 would be ten times as strong, with strength of one hundred (10 x 10). A pH of 4.0 compared to a pH of 7.0 would have strength of one thousand (10 x 10 x 10). Similarly, as a fluid pH moves upward on the scale, it increases exponentially in alkaline strength.

Healthy body cells are slightly alkaline. In disease states, cellular pH is below 6.8. The more acidic cells become, the sicker we are and can feel. Cells do not die until their pH falls to approximately 3.5, but in the process of getting there, many different disease symptoms can manifest. For instance, cancer begins to form at pH 5.5 due to deficient cellular oxygen.

The pH of saliva and urine upon waking are reliable indicators of acidity or alkalinity of body fluids and tissues. Saliva pH indicates the strength of the body's reserve of alkaline minerals stored in tissues and bones. pH of the first urine of the day is the main reflector of the present level of acidity or alkalinity of fluids within the body. It provides a picture of what the kidneys are attempting to eliminate. Minerals the body voids through urine are mainly the excess of either acid or alkaline water-soluble minerals. It gives an indication of whether we fed our body an acidifying diet or an alkalizing diet.

During the day the pH of both saliva and urine are influenced by what we eat and drink. Therefore, they will fluctuate. pH is also affected by our emotions. Stress and tension from negative emotions such as anger, worry, fear, resentment, jealousy, and stress are significant body acidifiers, causing a drain on our alkaline mineral reserves. Positive emotions and feelings such as love, gratitude, forgiveness, happiness, hope, and peace have an alkalizing effect in the body.

In perfect balance and health, both saliva and urine, upon waking, should be in the 6.8 to 7.2 range.

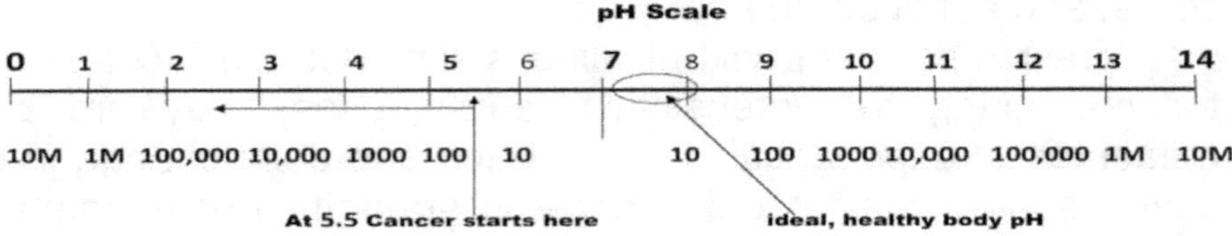

Internal fluids should be slightly alkaline for health. The easy way to measure this is with pH test strips, available online or in health food stores.

Checking your pH

URINE pH (first in the morning)

- Indicates pH of interstitial fluids in and around cells

- Also reflects recent, 24-hour, diet and lifestyle (foods, drinks, emotions)

- Should be between 6.8 and 7.2. (When hyper-alkalizing with sodium bicarbonate, readings should be between 7.2 and 8.4, or even up to 9.0)

SALIVA pH (first in the morning)

- Indicates strength of the body's alkaline mineral reserves – Sodium, calcium, magnesium, potassium, iron.

- Should be between 6.8 and 7.2

Purpose of the Alkaline Mineral Reserve

The body maintains an alkaline mineral reserve of sodium, calcium, potassium, magnesium, and iron in its tissues and bones. An overly-acidic diet and lifestyle has an acidifying effect on blood and plasma. In order to maintain blood pH at 7.365, the body withdraws alkaline minerals from its tissues to neutralize the acid condition and maintain health of the blood. As this withdrawal continues over time, tissues weaken, vitality lowers, and disease symptoms begin to appear.

Cholesterol is not the problem we have been told

Cholesterol is made by the body: 1. as its primary antacid, 2. to repair acid damage in tissues such as inside artery walls, and 3. to make hormones. Cholesterol lowering drugs work against body health.

A fat body is acidic

To protect internal organs from harm, the body stores excess acid residues in fat. On a balanced acid/alkaline diet, the body does not need to retain excess fat.

Note: When pH values are low and you embark on a dietary correction program, "the solution is to hyper-perfuse the blood and then the interstitial fluids with alkaline compounds of sodium and potassium bicarbonate." – Dr. Robert O Young

You can do this by drinking alkaline water with ½ to 1 tsp aluminum-free baking soda added, 3 or 4 times each day. During this period, urine pH should be between 7.2 and 8.4, or even up to 9.0.

When saliva pH is low, it can take some time on a correct diet to replenish the alkaline mineral reserve and to reflect this in first morning saliva pH readings. Be patient but persistent.

SECTION 9: How to alkalize and help your body

"Let food be your medicine, and let your medicine be food."
- Hippocrates

Avoid or minimize food and drinks that produce acids
- All animal products
- All dairy, including milk, cheese and eggs
- Alcohol and soft drinks
- Sugar, from any source
- Excess simple carbohydrates such as pasta, breads and baked goods, because they convert to sugar in the body
- Processed foods
- Read food labels to avoid toxic ingredients and chemical flavor enhancers
- Also Smoking, which is very harmful

About protein: It is a myth that we need lots of protein to build muscle. The body is 7% protein, while meats are 20 to 30% protein; *a large imbalance!* When we were babies we gained body tissue very quickly on mother's milk alone, which contains approximately 1% protein.

Excess protein produces acids that corrode tissues and lower body fluid pH, resulting in reduced levels of blood oxygen and energy. The strongest mammals on earth, such as the elephant, horse, and gorilla, eat no meat.

About sugar: Sugar, in all its forms, causes fermentation in the body, which leads to the growth of yeast, fungus, and reduced cellular oxygen levels. Fermentation produces alcohol with a pH of approximately 4.0.

Be aware of your emotions

- Negative emotions of anger, hate, fear, worry, and resentment are acid-producing
- Positive emotions of love, gratitude, forgiveness, hope, happiness, and peace are alkaline-producing

Maximize alkaline-producing foods in your diet

- Raw, ripe low-sweet fruits, berries, melons, and their fresh juices – preferably organic
- Raw vegetables and their fresh juices – preferably organic
  - ➤ Some of the best are: avocado, grapefruit, lemons, tomato, cucumber, celery, and dark green leafy vegetables
- Green smoothies made from a combination of fruits, berries and green leafy vegetables.
- Cooked vegetables, lightly steamed
- Alkaline grains – quinoa and millet
- Alkaline water
- Sodium bicarbonate (Aluminum-free baking soda)

Food Preparation

In order to consume a high percentage of food fresh and raw, this author recommends the regular use of a Vita-Mix blender and a juicer to prepare smoothies and juices.

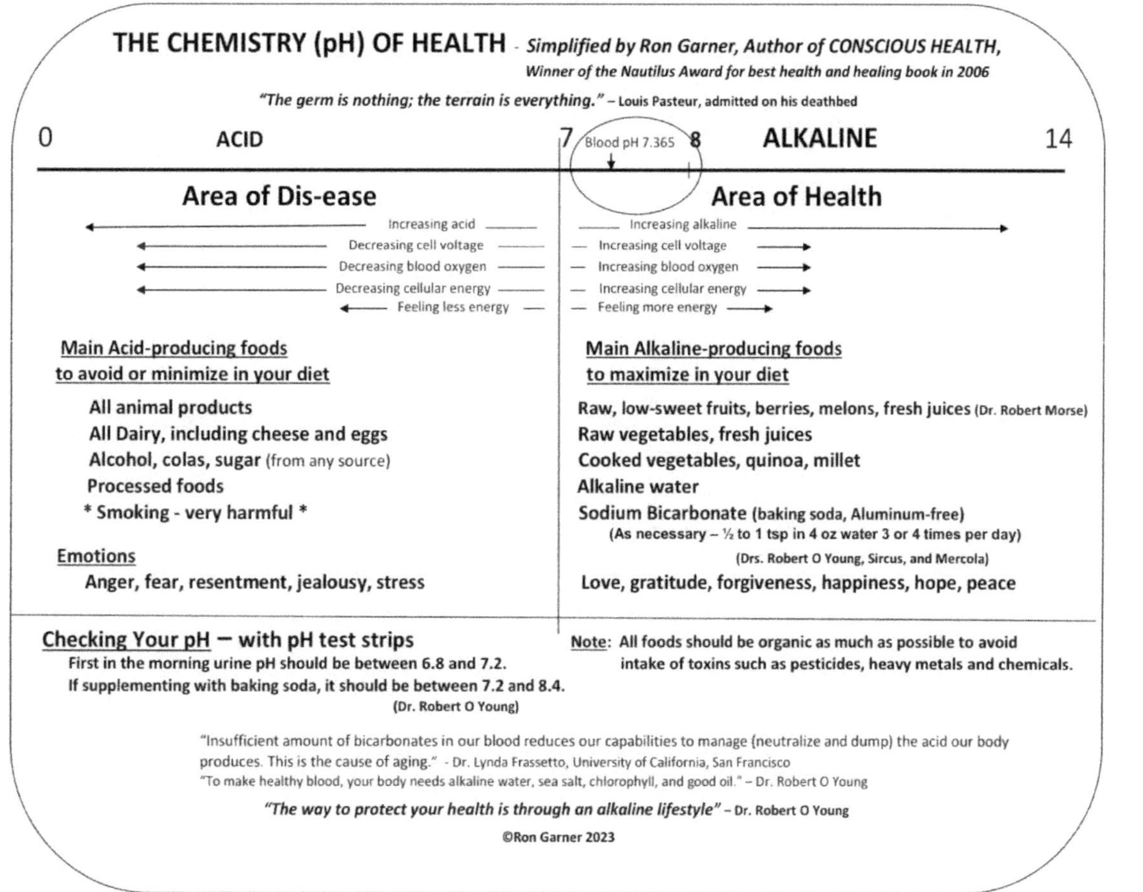

THE CHEMISTRY (pH) OF HEALTH - Simplified by Ron Garner, Author of CONSCIOUS HEALTH,
Winner of the Nautilus Award for best health and healing book in 2006

"The germ is nothing; the terrain is everything." – Louis Pasteur, admitted on his deathbed

0   ACID   7 Blood pH 7.365 8   ALKALINE   14

Area of Dis-ease   Area of Health

Increasing acid   Increasing alkaline
Decreasing cell voltage   Increasing cell voltage
Decreasing blood oxygen   Increasing blood oxygen
Decreasing cellular energy   Increasing cellular energy
Feeling less energy   Feeling more energy

Main Acid-producing foods
to avoid or minimize in your diet

All animal products
All Dairy, including cheese and eggs
Alcohol, colas, sugar (from any source)
Processed foods
* Smoking - very harmful *

Emotions
Anger, fear, resentment, jealousy, stress

Main Alkaline-producing foods
to maximize in your diet

Raw, low-sweet fruits, berries, melons, fresh juices (Dr. Robert Morse)
Raw vegetables, fresh juices
Cooked vegetables, quinoa, millet
Alkaline water
Sodium Bicarbonate (baking soda, Aluminum-free)
(As necessary – ½ to 1 tsp in 4 oz water 3 or 4 times per day)
(Drs. Robert O Young, Sircus, and Mercola)
Love, gratitude, forgiveness, happiness, hope, peace

Checking Your pH – with pH test strips
First in the morning urine pH should be between 6.8 and 7.2.
If supplementing with baking soda, it should be between 7.2 and 8.4.
(Dr. Robert O Young)

Note: All foods should be organic as much as possible to avoid
intake of toxins such as pesticides, heavy metals and chemicals.

"Insufficient amount of bicarbonates in our blood reduces our capabilities to manage (neutralize and dump) the acid our body
produces. This is the cause of aging." - Dr. Lynda Frassetto, University of California, San Francisco
"To make healthy blood, your body needs alkaline water, sea salt, chlorophyll, and good oil." – Dr. Robert O Young

"The way to protect your health is through an alkaline lifestyle" – Dr. Robert O Young

©Ron Garner 2023

 Why Blood Oxygen is Important and How to Increase it

Oxygen is the gas of health and energy. When oxygen levels in the body are lower than normal, organisms such as bacteria, parasites, yeast, and fungus begin to thrive and transform. This leads to disease.

Cells normally produce energy by using oxygen. As acidification increases in the body and less oxygen is available, energy production in cells shifts from using an aerobic (oxygen) process to using an anaerobic (lack of oxygen) fermentation process. This results in a ten-fold decrease of energy production. The more acidic the body becomes the faster disease organisms can multiply.

A Good Example of Serious Acidosis is Cancer

When the pH of tissues declines to 5.5, cancer starts to grow. In the 1930's Dr. Otto Warburg discovered that cancer cannot live in the presence of oxygen. He stated: "The fundamental cause of *all degenerative disease* is hypoxia; oxygen starvation at the cellular level."

Dr. Robert Morse states: "Cancer doesn't just suddenly appear in the body. By the time you see cancer in one place, you are lymphatically backed up from head to toe. Cancer doesn't move. The systemic acids are simply burning and mutating cells in other areas." Killing cancer in one place with radiation or chemotherapy does not correct the systemic acidosis problem that allowed cancer to begin in the first place. The basic cause, lack of oxygen, must be addressed for permanent elimination of cancer to be achieved.

Consider an Analogy

If you are trying to extinguish a fire that was started with gasoline, would you continue to put more gasoline on the fire? Absolutely not!

So…if you are trying to reverse a health condition that was caused by acid buildup in tissues, would it make sense to continue the same diet of acid-producing foods you had been eating before? How would this increase blood oxygen levels? Of course, it would not.

Kind of a no-brainer, don't you think?

How to increase blood oxygen levels:
1. Shift to a more-alkaline diet
2. Work to increase urine and saliva pH
3. Supplement 3 or 4 times daily with ½ to 1 tsp of aluminum-free baking soda in a glass of clean, filtered water
4. Practice deep breathing
5. Exercise moderately but regularly
6. Bath soaks in very warm water with one or a combination of sea salt, Epsom salts, and/or baking soda added.
7. Bath soaks with food grade hydrogen peroxide added.
8. In some cases of serious health conditions - hyperbaric oxygen treatments to quickly but temporarily boost oxygen levels in the body.

There are three main tools the author uses to monitor his health status and progress on a regular basis:

1. **pH Testing**
   Urine pH (first in the morning)
   - Indicates pH of interstitial fluids in and around cells
   - Should be between 6.8 and 7.2. (When hyper-profusing with sodium bicarbonate, readings should be between 7.2 and 8.4, or even up to 9.0.)

   Saliva pH (first in the morning)
   - Indicates strength of the body's alkaline mineral reserves
   - Should be between 6.8 and 7.2

2. **Blood Pressure Monitor**
   (From Dr. Robert Morse's Detox Miracle Sourcebook)

   - Blood pressure readings (both arms) – The first number (systolic) is adrenal strength. The second number (diastolic) indicates kidney efficiency. The ideal is 120-130 / 60-70. This number indicates that the adrenals are strong, and the kidneys are filtering properly with no resistance.

   - High blood pressure – "begins when the kidneys start to go down." It is caused by congested kidneys, weak adrenals, lymphatic congestion, and loss of calcium, weakening the vascular system. "All high blood pressure cases are actually low blood pressure because the kidneys and adrenals are involved." "…when the bodies are detoxified, then blood pressure will reflect this."

   - Low blood pressure – is related to weak adrenal glands.

Comment: I find blood pressure readings to be very helpful, along with checking my urine for sediment. They show me how I am progressing, and what I should be working on to strengthen my adrenal gland and kidney functions.

3. Oximeter – to test blood oxygen content

SECTION 13:   How the Body Heals

The body heals naturally and in definite stages *when* it has accumulated sufficient nutrition and energy above and beyond basic living requirements.

In Order of Priority

Considering that the body's first priority is to stay alive, its first healing efforts will be directed to parts of the body most vital to survival.

In Cycles

The body works on each priority area until it is no longer the highest, moving on to the next worst condition after that. Little by little, vitality is raised and overall health is improved. As conditions improve in each area, the body will cycle back again to work on areas that are partially healed, to increase health levels further. This way, it gradually works toward complete health, but of course this takes time.

When the intake of healthy food is greater than the intake of unhealthy food, the balance is tipped in favor of the body; it is able to divert some of its efforts away from survival toward healing. After a period of time on a nutritious alkaline diet, the body will be ready to do some serious detoxification and will bring on what is called a healing crisis, such as a cold or flu. It follows a clear pattern in the process of healing itself. The most serious and most recent disease conditions are given first attention. As progress is made on these, the body works backwards in time, so to speak, retracing and correcting other conditions in reverse order to when they appeared. Remember that this is all conditional on the body continuing to receive regular nutrition and rest, over and above that which is required to carry on daily activities, so it doesn't have to borrow from its own stored reserves to accomplish the process.

The body cannot complete the tasks of serious detoxification and healing and still provide energy for everyday activities. Rest is required. That is why we feel tired during a cold or flu. These are times of intense internal cleansing. The body doesn't have less energy; it is redirecting the energy it does have for internal healing purposes.

We may continue to experience periods of illness and low energy during these cycles. However, during a healing crisis, there is one very large difference. This time, under the influence of a healthy lifestyle, the body experiences symptoms related to a disease *healing* crisis, as opposed to a disease *survival* crisis. At the completion of such a crisis, the body will have *gained* vitality, not *lost* vitality. The body is getting stronger, not weaker.

The healthier we become, the less intense and often healing crises will be.

The new biology of digestion

Dr. Robert O Young, author of *The pH Miracle*, has worked for more than 40 years examining various body fluids using high-magnification microscopy. The results of his research resulted in some surprising findings regarding how food is processed in the body. Contrary to conventional medical thinking, he discovered:

1. **The importance of sodium bicarbonate**

     As food is chewed in the mouth, sodium bicarbonate is secreted by the salivary glands. When food reaches the stomach, more sodium bicarbonate is added. Finally, as the now liquefied food (chyme) moves into the small intestine, if further alkalinity is needed, additional sodium bicarbonate is secreted by the pancreas to bring the pH to 8.4.

2. **The stomach is an organ of contribution, not digestion**

     The stomach combines salt, water, and carbon dioxide to produce sodium bicarbonate and hydrochloric acid.

$$NaCl + H_2O + CO_2 \longrightarrow NaHCO_3 + HCl$$

     Sodium bicarbonate is what is needed. Hydrochloric acid is waste that must be eliminated. Hydrochloric acid falls to the bottom of the stomach where it is transported via fascia tissues throughout the body to be eliminated by perspiration, respiration, urination, defecation, and in women – also by menstruation.

3. **Blood cells are created in the crypts of the small intestine**

     The main purpose of chyme processing at pH 8.4 in the small intestine is to create stem cells and new blood cells.

4. **Nutrients needed to create healthy blood**

     Healthy blood is created from chlorophyll, oil, salt, and water. That is why it is so important to eat raw green leafy vegetables, sea salt, and natural oil such as coconut, avocado, flax and fish oil.

The body's great lymphatic system

As taught by Dr. Robert Morse, acid wastes are eliminated from cells into the interstitial fluid that surrounds them – the lymphatic fluid system. This waste matter is then transported to and through the kidneys to be filtered and eliminated in urine. Again, contrary to conventional medical thinking, this is why urine should contain fine particles or sediment, and not always be clear. Evidence of sediment indicates that the kidneys are functioning properly.

Always remember

All pain, except from direct physical injury, is caused by acidosis. Acids are corrosive; they burn tissues. Burning is painful. The remedy for all disease symptoms is *always* alkalization and detoxification. Keep working to alkalize and clear lymphatic congestion.

SECTION 15:   Words of Encouragement

You've just finished the foundational part of this natural health book/course and you may be thinking, "This is too much change all at once for me; it's too overwhelming and I don't want to give up all the foods I like" etc., etc. But don't let that stop you from doing something. The renewed energy and feelings of positive well-being are so worth it.

Remember the 80/20 rule

The 80/20 rule, also known as the Pareto Principle, is usually applied to business and economics. It states that *80% of consequences come from 20% of the causes.*

Now, if we apply this principle to health, we can conclude that: *If you do 80% of things right, the other 20% can probably be handled by your body.* In other words, you don't have to be perfect to make gains, unless you are fighting a life-threatening disease condition in which case maximum efforts need be made.

So don't just give up. Start removing the worst things from your diet one by one. Then gradually move toward more healthy diet and lifestyle choices as time moves on.

Your body always wants to be healthy

Only you can determine the level of faith you put into this knowledge and the level of commitment you put into applying it to your life. The final decisions are always yours. Life is all about choices. Your body always works to produce health as long as you give it the tools it needs.

Don't lose sleep over a doctor's diagnosis, because it is nothing but confirmation of yesterday's poor choices. Instead, focus on today and tomorrow will be yours.

NEVER GIVE UP

THERE IS ALWAYS HOPE!

Give someone a fish and you feed them for a day.
Teach them to fish and they eat for a lifetime.

In the lessons of this book/course you have been given (fed) the main key understandings for creating a healthy body. But by learning how to search for information yourself, you become a knowledgeable, continuous thinker and decision-maker regarding what to do about taking responsibility for your own health. You depend much less on others for new information.

There is a vast amount of information available on the Internet; you only need to know what to look for and search for it. Just remember that your body was made to function in harmony with nature – natural foods, herbs, supplements, and energies, not synthetic chemicals and processed foods. Accordingly, look for information from naturally-oriented health sources, and depend less on medical and pharmaceutically-based information. Learn to ask yourself questions! Not everything we are told to do by health authorities is *safe and effective!*

For example, before taking a drug that is being prescribed for you, check online to find out what its ingredients are, what it is sourced from, and what its side effects are – can it cause stress or injury to organs in your body?

Another example would be foods and supplements – are they grown organically, do they contain pesticides or poisonous sprays, do they contain harmful ingredients such as heavy metals, have they been processed and if so how?

It's not what you think you know that's
most important…it's the questions you ask.

Example topics to start searching:

- Definition of words you don't understand
- Why dental infections can hold back healing in other parts of the body (Teeth are connected to acupuncture meridians throughout the body.)

- The downside of root canals (When the root nerve is removed, the tooth dies and has no natural circulation for defense from harmful bacteria.)
- The danger of fluoride
- What drugs can cause damage to kidneys, liver, heart, glands, etc.
- What drugs or injections can cause myocarditis
- What can dissolve blood clots
- Why everyone needs iodine (On average, North Americans are very deficient in Iodine.)
- Liver cleansing best methods (The liver performs more than 500 functions in the body.)
- Oils needed for healthy cell membranes (eg. Why canola oil and other seed oils are harmful)
- Why deep fried foods are harmful
- The most heat-tolerant oils for cooking
- Words used on ingredient labels to mask MSG (monosodium glutamate), which is used as a flavor enhancer, but is also a potent neurotoxin
- What is the purpose of diarrhea or a fever (The body does everything for a reason and nothing by accident. It doesn't attack itself, as in "auto-immune")

The above are only a few items to get you started on your path to being inquisitive and practiced in finding answers on your own. You are capable of taking major control of your future health by gaining information you need. It all starts with your decision to do it and thinking for yourself.

SECTION 17: **Self-Test**

How well do you understand the material you have just read? Could you explain the main principles to others? To test your grasp of this knowledge, see if you can answer the following questions. Then, you can quickly re-read sections to refresh and reinforce the important information in your memory.

1. What was the purpose of the Flexner Report?
2. What is the difference between allopathic and naturopathic modes of healing?
3. What is disease?
4. What was the original meaning of 'doctor'?
5. What is the main cause of disease?
6. Why do disease symptoms develop?
7. How does cancer begin, and does it remain in one area of the body? Why?
8. Explain why health is simple to understand.
9. Explain the pH scale to yourself or someone else.
10. Explain the new understanding of digestion.
11. Explain the process the body goes through when healing.
12. What is the pH of healthy blood and why is it important to maintain?
13. What are the healthy ranges for urine and saliva pH readings and what do they mean?
14. How are body fluid pH and cellular voltage related?
15. How can we increase energy (cellular voltage)?
16. State some examples of electron donors and electron stealers.

17. What effect do positive and negative emotions have on acid/alkaline balance?
18. What are the most important organs of detoxification?

19. What are the two main sources of acid production in the body?
20. Why do colds and flues happen?
21. Why does a body retain excess fat?
22. What is a healing crisis?
23. What are some effective means to help the body detoxify?
24. What is dry fasting, and why is it effective?
25. What are the main acid-producing foods?
26. What are the main alkaline-producing foods?
27. What advantages do organic foods have over non-organic foods?
28. Why should we read food labels?
29. What is the purpose of supplementing with aluminum-free baking soda?
30. How can you monitor your health progress?

MAIN FACTS TO REMEMBER

The stomach is an organ of contribution, not digestion
1. Sodium bicarbonate is produced to alkalize food
2. Hydrochloric acid is also produced as a bi-product waste that must be eliminated

Top alkaline foods to eat often - raw
1. Cucumber
2. Tomato
3. Avocado
4. Celery
5. Salad greens
6. Almonds – soaked overnight
7. Sprouted seeds
8. Grapefruit – low sweet
9. Lemons, limes – ripe (slightly soft)

To make healthy blood your body needs: C O W S
1. Chlorophyll – from green vegetables, and green grass powders such as alfalfa, barley, wheat
2. Oil – hemp, flax, olive, coconut, fish, Udo's. (No processed vegetable oils)
3. Water - alkaline
4. Salt (sea) – Himalayan, Celtic. (Not table salt)

Tools to monitor your health indications
1. pH test strips
2. Blood pressure monitor
3. Body temperature thermometer

4. Oximeter
5. Notebook to record your progress

To speed up alkalizing interstitial fluids (Super- perfusing)

Aluminum-free baking soda (Sodium Bicarbonate): ½ to 1 tsp in glass of water 3 or 4 times per day.
Urine pH should be between 7.2 and 8.4. (Even to 9.0)

How to have a strong immune system and avoid disease

Maintain the alkaline design of your body.

Foods to Eat Freely

The pH Miracle Alkaline-Acid Food Chart

Copyright 2013 – pH Miracle Inc.

Mildly Alkaline	Moderately Alkaline	Highly Alkaline
Almond Milk	Fresh Coconut Water	pH 9.5 Water
Distilled Water		Green Drinks
	Arugula	
Artichokes	Beets	Himalayan Salt
Asparagus	Basil	Real Salt
Brussels Sprouts	Capsicum/Pepper	
Cauliflower	Cabbage Lettuce	Avocado
Comfrey	Carrot	Broccoli
Kohlrabi	Chives	Cabbage
Lamb's Lettuce	Collard/Spring Greens	Celery
Leeks	Coriander	Cucumber
New Baby Potatoes	Endive	Endive
Peas	Ginger	Garlic
Pumpkin	Green Beans	Grasses (alfalfa, bean, pea, soy, etc.)
Onion	Leeks	Spinach
Rutabaga	Lettuce	
Swede	Mustard Greens	
Squash (Butternut, Summer, etc.)	Okra	Soy Nuts
Watercress	Radish	(soaked soybeans, then air-dried)
White Cabbage	Red Cabbage	
		Soy Lecithin, pure

Mildly Alkaline	**Moderately Alkaline**
Coconut	Red Onion
Grapefruit	Turnip
Pomegranate	Zucchini
Almonds	Lemon
Fennel Seeds	Lime
Lentils	Rhubarb
Tofu	
Sesame Seeds	Butter Beans
	Lima Beans
Herbs & Spices	Soy Beans (Fresh)
	White (Navy) Beans
Avocado Oil	
Olive Oil	Chia/Salba Seeds
Coconut Oil	Hemp Seeds
Flax Oil	Quinoa
Grapeseed Oil	
Hemp Oil	
pH Miracle Omega 3-6-9 Oil	

The pH Miracle Alkaline-Acid Food Chart

Copyright 2013 – pH Miracle Inc.

Highly Acidic	**Moderately Acidic**	**Mildly Acidic**
Alcohol	Fresh, Natural Juice	Rice, Soy & Coconut Milk
Coffee & Black Tea		
Fruit Juice (Sweetened)	Ketchup	Cantaloupe
	Mayonnaise	Fresh Dates
Cocoa	Butter	Nectarine
Honey Jam		Plum
Jelly	Apple	Sweet Cherry
Mustard	Apricot	Watermelon
Miso	Banana	
Rice Syrup	Blackberry	Black Beans
Vinegar	Blueberry	Garbanzo Beans
Yeast	Cranberry	Kidney Beans
	Grapes	Seitan
Dried Fruit	Guava	
	Mango	Aramanth
Beef	Mangosteen	Buckwheat Groats
Chicken	Orange	Buckwheat Pasta
Eggs	Peach	Millet
Farmed Fish	Papaya	Oats/Oatmeal

Highly Acidic	**Moderately Acidic**	**Mildly Acidic**
Pork	Pineapple	Soybeans
Shellfish	Strawberry	Spelt
		Cous Cous
White Rice	Goat's Cheese	
Cheese	Vegan Cheese	Rice/Soy/Hemp Protein
Dairy		
	Brown Rice	Freshwater Wild fish
Artificial Sweeteners	Rye Bread	
Syrup	Wheat	Brazil Nuts
	Wholemeal Bread	Flax Seeds
Mushroom	Wild Rice	Hazelnuts
	Wholemeal Pasta	Macadamia Nuts
		Pecans
	Walnuts	Pumpkin Seeds
		Sumflower Seeds
	Ocean Fish	
		Sunflower Oil

pH Interpretation (Dr. Robert O Young)

pH – The pH of the body has a profound effect on the inner environment and the microscopic organisms in the body. The pH of blood and tissues should be approximately 7.365. The pH of saliva should be 6.8 to 7.2.

> (Note by Ron Garner) – When one starts to hyper-alkalize to correct over-acidity, urine pH will indicate above 7.2. Healthy first in morning saliva readings can take quite a while to move upwards into the alkaline range.)

Urine

- Urine pH is a measurement of the interstitial fluids of the Interstitium.
- First in the morning – indicates pH of body tissues. Healthy urine pH should be in the 7.2 or greater range. But there are broad swings in this pH, depending on what you have been drinking in the last 24 hours.
  (People who have to get up at night to urinate do so because their bodies need to reduce the acid load from their body tissues)
- When you work to raise/normalize pH, by alkalization and hyper-alkalization, the urine pH will gradually rise.
- Saliva, urine, sweat, and tears pH should measure at least 7.2. "If you maintain your saliva and urine pH at 7.2 or above, you will never get sick!"
- When your muscles are sore, that's the tissues picking up the acid to maintain the blood pH. When the lymphatic system is healthy it will pull the lactic acid out of the tissues, and eventually you will sweat it out or it will be recycled back into the blood and you will urinate it out.

Saliva

- When you are testing your saliva, you are testing your ability or potential to alkalize your food and drink. ie. Your body's alkaline reserves.

Interstitium (fascia tissues) - fluid-filled spaces in connective tissues all over the body, including below the skin's surface; lining the digestive tract, lungs and urinary systems, and surrounding muscles.
The interstitial fluids are the fluid areas that surround every cell of the body and hold alkalinity or electrons for cellular energy and acidic wastes that are waiting to be removed by the lymphatic system through the four channels of elimination (perspiration, urination, defecation, and respiration). They are the acid-catchers of the blood and body cells and are at an ideal pH of 7.2.

Obesity – is the way the body reacts to indulgence of foods that create excess fermentation and acids. The body retains fat in order to bind the dietary and metabolic acids away from the organs that sustain life.

Cancer - is a systemic acidic problem that has localized in the weakest parts of the body. Cancer begins at pH 5.5.

Microform Bacteria
Transform from bacteria to yeast to fungus and finally mould in the body due to prolonged acidity of fluids and tissues. Overgrowth leads to all disease forms such athlete's foot, Candida, diabetes, cancer, atherosclerosis, osteoporosis, chronic fatigue, etc. The wastes they produce are strong acids.

Even at serious disease states, these conditions can be reversed by creating an internal alkaline environment in the body that will not support the transformation and development of microforms. Needed is alkalizing the blood and tissue pH with appropriate nutritional supplements and an alkaline lifestyle and diet.

Sugar
"Sugar is a metabolic acidic waste and should never be ingested in any form without serious health consequences!" All sugars ferment and provide fuel for Candida and

microform bacteria to produce energy for them to live. Acetyl alcohol is a by-product of yeast's sugar fermentation and is very damaging to body cells.

Diet of most people

pH of Typical Diet

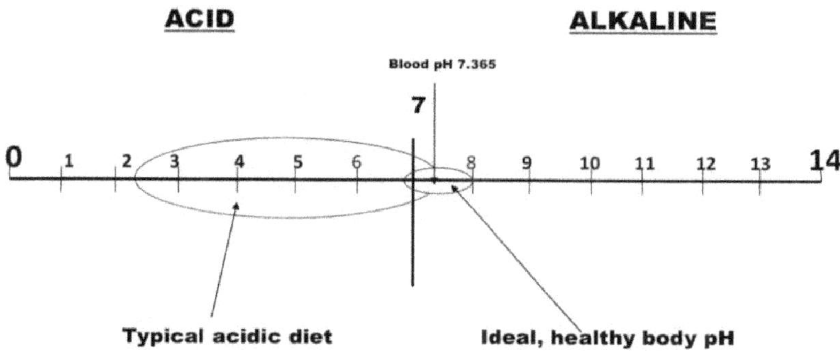

Notice that the typical diet of most people overbalances healthy body pH by approximately 1000 to 1, acid to alkaline. This causes a steady depletion of alkaline minerals from body tissues and bones in order to maintain healthy blood pH. Over time, as tissues become more acidic, a decrease in cellular voltage, oxygen, and energy result. As this continues, disease symptoms begin to appear and worsen unless pH balance is restored to the body.

pH of Various Liquids

<u>pH of Typical liquids</u>		<u>Times more acidic than water at pH 7</u>
ACID DRINKS		
❖ wine	3 to 4	1,000 to 10,000
❖ beer	3.2 to 5.3	70 to 10,000
❖ cider	2.9 to 3.3	10,000
❖ champagne	2.9	10,000
❖ vodka	4 to 7	Neutral to 1000
❖ whisky	3.5 to 5	100 to 5000
❖ gin	6 to 7	Neutral to 10
❖ kombucha tea	2.4 to 4.5	500 to 60,000
❖ Pellegrino	5.3	70
❖ Sparkling thirsty Buddha	4.4	600
❖ Coca Cola	2.4	60,000
❖ Milk 2%	6.6	4
❖ Green tea	7	Neutral
❖ Black tea	5 to 5.5	15 to 100
❖ Coffee	5	100
❖ Orange juice	3.3 to 4.2	2,000 to 10,000
❖ Vinegar	2 to 3	10,000 to 100,000
ACIDS		
❖ Ascorbic acid (is not complete Vit C)	3	10,000
❖ Lactic acid	3.5	5000
❖ Acetic acid	4	1,000
❖ Carbonic acid	4 to 5	100 to 1000
❖ Hydrochloric acid	1 to 3	10,000 TO 1M
❖ Nitric acid	1 to 3	10,000 TO 1M
❖ Sulfuric acid	1 to 3	10,000 TO 1M
❖ Phosphoric acid	1 to 2	100,000 TO 1M

ALKALINE LIQUIDS

- ❖ Tap water   7.0 average or less
  depends on source and additives)
- ❖ Bottled spring water (green)   7.6
- ❖ Ionized water (Ionizer)   7 to 11
- ❖ Ocean water   8.4
- ❖ Baking soda   8
- ❖ Household ammonia   11
- ❖ Household bleach   12

* Raw ripe lemon, lime, grapefruit – are acidic but leave an alkaline residue in the body.

Excerpts from YouTube Teachings of Dr. Robert Morse (rawfigs.com)

Reference sources are in brackets, indicating the number or name of the Q&A Video where it was found. Please note there may be other videos by Dr. Morse where the same subject is discussed.

- **Adrenal glands** – control the kidneys and mineral utilization in the body, and play a role in sugar metabolism, body shape and size. They produce steroids, which are responsible for utilization of minerals and nutrients in food, as well as hormones (cortisol, progesterone, estrogen, and testosterone). When the adrenals are weak, the kidneys become weak and the myelin sheath of nerves also become weaker, which can affect the entire neurological system. The adrenals control the autonomic nervous system – energy, breathing, heart pumping, peristalsis. (310, 227, 230)

- **Anxiety and panic attacks** – are caused from a backed-up lymphatic system, weak adrenals, and low production of neurotransmitters. These conditions are made worse by neurotoxins in foods and in the home environment. Detoxification is needed to move lymph, clean and strengthen kidneys, adrenals, and the transverse colon. (45 Part 2, 252)

- **Arthritis** – is caused by inflammation (acidity) in the joints, but also indicates that acidosis is affecting the entire body. If you try to treat it as a 'disease,' this will not correct the cause. (65 Part 2, 158)

- **Autoimmune problem** – There is no such thing! It is an allopathic concept to describe something they don't understand and leads us to believe it is something that cannot be understood or corrected. Your body does not create its own problems. It never makes a mistake and does everything for a reason – to cope with the situation it is forced to deal with, which involves breaking down and removing damaged cells because they have become part of the problem. Remember the rule of nature is the weak perish and the strong survive. What doctors call autoimmune is part of the natural process of discarding weakness so it can be replaced and rebuilt with strength. But, of course, that depends on the body being detoxified and supplied with the nutrition it needs to do this. (32 Part 3, 75 Part 1, 86, Part 1)

- **Bacterial infections** – Bacteria are part of nature's clean-up crew. They come into areas of toxic overload to eat and neutralize toxins in the lymph fluid. Antibiotics kill bacteria but do nothing about the basic problem – toxic lymph.

- **Beef, pork, fowl meats, fish, dairy products, cheese** – are stimulants and too high in protein content.

- **Blood pressure readings (both arms)** – The first number (systolic) is adrenal strength. The second number (diastolic) indicates kidney efficiency. Ideal is 120-130/60-70. This number indicates that the adrenals are strong, and the kidneys are filtering properly with no resistance. The systolic reading is a reflection of epinephrine and nor-epinephrine being produced by the adrenal glands. These are neurotransmitters that pump the heart. (Detox Miracle Sourcebook p. 45)

  - **High** – "begins when the kidneys start to go down." It is caused by congested kidneys, weak adrenals, lymphatic congestion, and loss of calcium weakening the vascular system. "All high blood pressure cases are actually low blood pressure because the kidneys and adrenals are involved." "…when the bodies are detoxified, then blood pressure will reflect this." (118 Part 2, 204, 290, Detox Miracle Sourcebook p.201)

  - **Low** – is related to weak adrenal glands. (82 Part 4)

  - **Swinging (fluctuating between high and low)** – is caused by lymphatic congestion in the cerebellum area of the brain. (132, 290)

- **Blood tests** – give only a fractional truth of what is going on in the body. They show nothing about the lymph, which is the major part of cellular fluid. (Indiana Talk Part 1)

- **Bowel movements, stinky** – are caused by protein putrefaction and toxemia. If you stink, you are getting rid of proteins – dead tissue in your body. Detoxification is needed. A fruit and vegetable diet does not cause this kind of odor. However, even on a strict fruit and vegetable diet, but after a cleansing fast, such as a dry fast, bowel movements can smell very bad due to deep cleansing of stored proteins and sulfur. (17 Part 6)

- **Cancer** – is not a disease (this is allopathic thinking); it is extreme acidosis in the genetically weak area of the body affected. Cancer cells are mutated cells damaged from acids in stagnant lymphatic fluid. The greatest food offender causing this kind of damage is dairy products. All cancers start with the kidneys not being able to filter and eliminate lymphatic wastes. "By the time you see cancer in one place, you are lymphatically backed up from head to toe. … Cancer doesn't move, the systemic acids are simply burning and mutating cells in other areas."(180) The solution, as in all cases of illness (acidosis), is alkalization and detoxification. Work on the thymus gland to improve immune response and help to move sluggish lymph flow. "Dr. Morse's clinic claims a 95% success rate in returning the body to a state of true health."[i] "When you have cancer you have one system down, and that is the lymphatic system." (For a brief easy-to-understand explanation of cancer, listen to video "55 Part 6". For a more detailed explanation, listen to: "Cancer – The Forbidden Cures".) (46 Part 2, 55 Part 6, 144, 240, 254, 285)

- **Cholesterol** – is the body's main lipid and antacid system. It is also used to repair vascular walls weakened from acid corrosion. There is no bad cholesterol, just two types of cholesterol used differently in the body. LDL is used predominantly to neutralize acids and HDL is used mainly in cell walls. Blood serum cholesterol has nothing to do with what the body is doing with cholesterol. You cannot suppress the body's production of cholesterol when it is using cholesterol as an antacid. Cholesterol is not the problem; it is systemic acidosis caused from eating too many acid-producing foods. Adrenals and kidneys must be strengthened to detoxify lymphatic acid wastes and bring body chemistry back into balance. (1 Part 1, 54 Part 4, 144)

- **Dairy products and cheese** – are extreme fungal foods and are mucus-forming. They congest the lymph, kidneys, and adrenals, and are the worst foods leading toward cancer. They are most congestive to the upper respiratory areas - throat, sinus. (199, 234, 236)

- **Fasting** – can be very powerful but needs to be worked up to slowly. In the opinion of the author, the following fasting modes are listed in order of increasing detoxification aggressiveness:

  o Freshly made raw fruit juice.
  o Mono-fruit eating. "The two best fruit fasts are lemon juice and dark grapes." (46 Part 4)
  o Intermittent dry fasting.
  o Water fasting.
  o Extended dry fasting.

- **Fermented foods** - are fungal foods on the decaying side of life. They create bloating, gas, and fungus in the body. (ATDCPRH, 135)

- **Fungus** – is formed during fermentation of carbohydrates. It leaves uric acid crystals in the body, especially in the presence of sulfur, because sulfur is a fungal proliferant. (3 Part 3)

- **Grains** – are dormant, concentrated foods containing complex sugars and enzyme inhibitors. The polysaccharide sugars feed fungus and parasites, require insulin to be utilized, and keep fat on the body. Grains are not healthy foods. Farmers don't feed grain to their meat animals except to fatten them up before slaughter. Sprouted grains are better. (7 Part 7, 14 Part 7, 119 Part 2, 201)

- **Healing progress** – is slow when kidney lymph filtration is poor. (68 Part 4)

- **Inflammation** – is another word for acidosis; it is an immune response to acid. Stagnation of lymph causes inflammation. Inflammation equals loss of calcium equals nerve spasms (and headaches). Need lymph drainage, strengthen adrenals and kidneys to reduce lymphatic congestion. (229, 290, 306, International School of Detoxification 4-28-2014)

- **Kidneys** – are vital eliminative organs of the lymphatic system, central to elimination of lymphatic wastes. (150)

- **Sleep problems** – are related to lymph stagnation in the pineal gland. A clean body needs about six or seven hours of sleep each night. If one wakes tired in the morning, work is needed to strengthen the adrenal, and thyroid glands to increase natural production of neurotransmitters. Also know that EMF radiation from Wi-Fi and electronic devices can depress the body's production of melatonin, which is your body's hormone that promotes sleep, among other important functions. Turning the Wi-Fi off at night gives your body a chance to rest, rejuvenate, and regenerate. (124 Part 1)

FOR MORE INFORMATION

There is a tremendous amount of information available on the Internet but the main problem is finding the most helpful; recognizing the difference between natural health and pharmaceutically-biased sources.

Following are some of the most helpful and leading-edge sources for natural health information this author has found:

Dr. Robert O Young, DSc, PhD - drrobertyoung.com
– Author of *The pH Miracle*

In my opinion, Dr. Young is one of the most brilliant and courageous doctors of our time. He is on the leading edge of research and development for information and supplements to counteract the harmful effects of air, water, food, needle injection toxins, and 5G, plus electromagnetic radiation we are forced to deal with in these present times.

Dr. Robert Morse, ND, DSc – drmorseherbalhealthclub.com

Dr. Morse's search engine: rawfigs.com - Type in any word topic you want to know more about and it will take you to a video clip of Dr. Morse answering similar questions from his clients.

Dr. Edward Group, DC – drgroup.com

Dr. Group founded Global Healing to help customers achieve optimum health and wellness through clean eating and nutritional supplementation. He is an expert authority on liver cleansing and urotherapy.

Dr. Bryan Ardis, DC – thedrardisshow.com

Dr. Ardis was the first doctor to solve the pandemic riddle, as he discovered the role of poisonous snake and sea cone venoms in some recommended injections.

Dr. Jerry Tennant, MD – tennantinstitute.com

Dr. Tennant is a world-renowned physician, author, and inventor who has made significant contributions to the field of integrative medicine. His work focuses on the concept of voltage and its role in cellular health, regeneration, and disease prevention. He is the author of *Healing is Voltage*.

Awakening to Health Website, including video clips of Ron Garner teaching:

http://www.awakeningtohealth.ca

INDEX